Lainy's

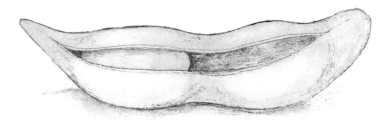

Polite Bite

Emma J. Fogt
Illustrated by Lori B. Wicks

ISBN 978-0-9913786-0-9

For my all: Franz, Tatiana and Tristan. EJF

For my sunshine: Dylan. LBW

Thank you Carrie Mark for
making this book a reality.

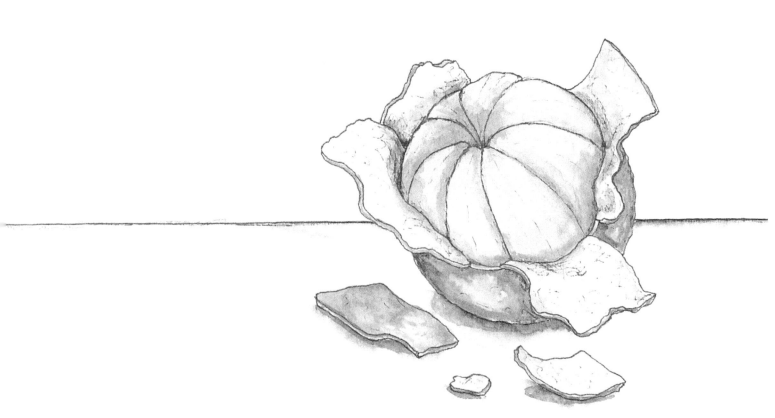

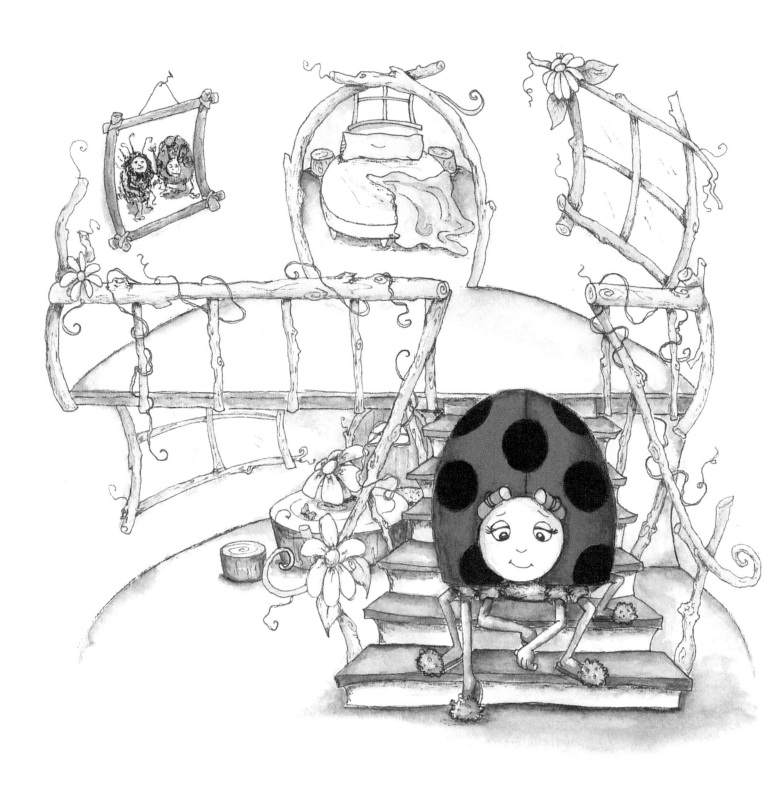

Lainy Ladybug woke up one morning and crawled
downstairs to the kitchen.

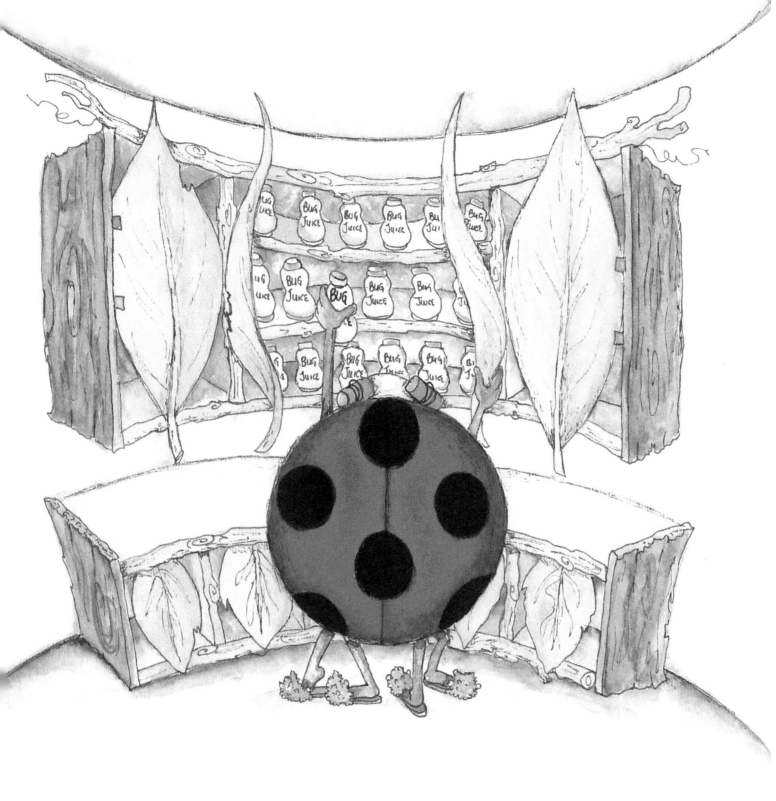

She peered into her cupboard and pulled out her all-time favorite breakfast: a little bottle of Bug Juice. Lainy enjoyed Bug Juice. It was cool and sweet.

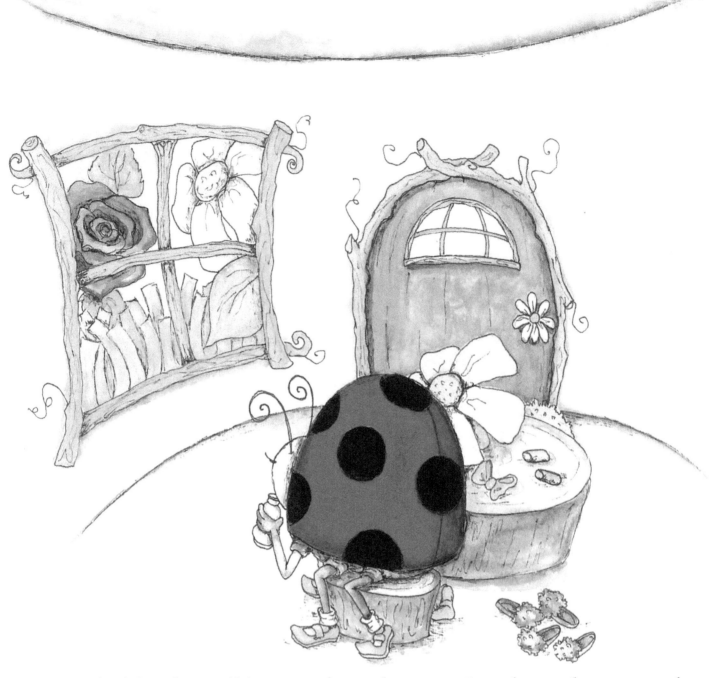

"Looks like this will hit just the right spots!" exclaimed Lainy with glee. As she drank her breakfast Lainy gazed dreamily out of her open window, while humming a little tune:

(Sung to: Row Row Row Your Boat)

Bug Juice, Bug Juice
It's my favorite treat
It's sweet and fresh
And tastes the best
It's all I want to eat

Snap Snap!

Slurp Slurp!

Slurrrrrrrrp!

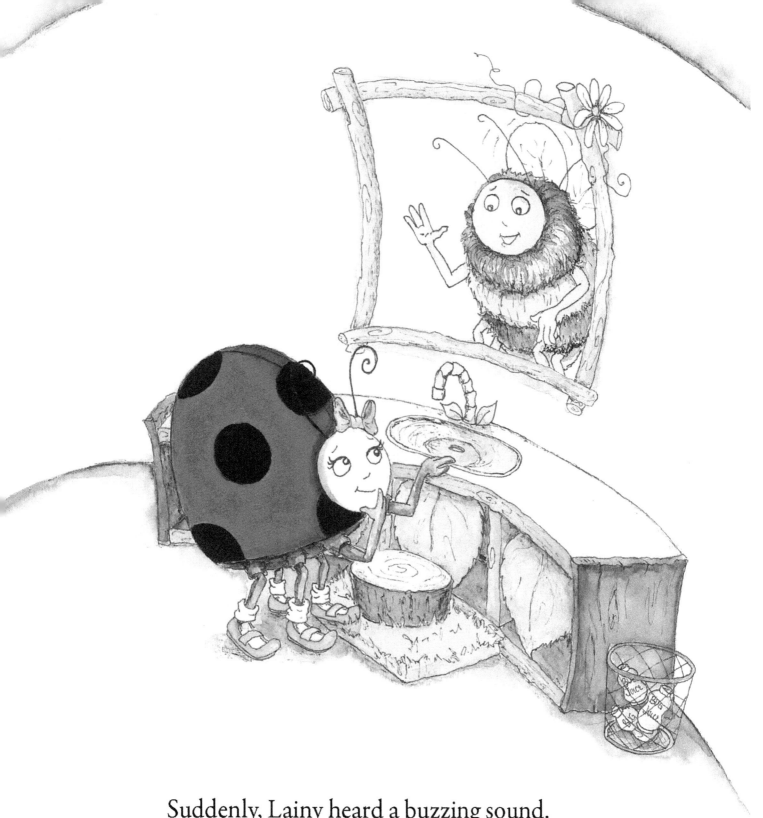

Suddenly, Lainy heard a buzzing sound.
Who whizzed by but her best friend, Benny Bumblebee.
"Good Morning Lainy! I was wondering if you would buzz on up
to The Farm with me today. It's such a lovely, sunny morning."

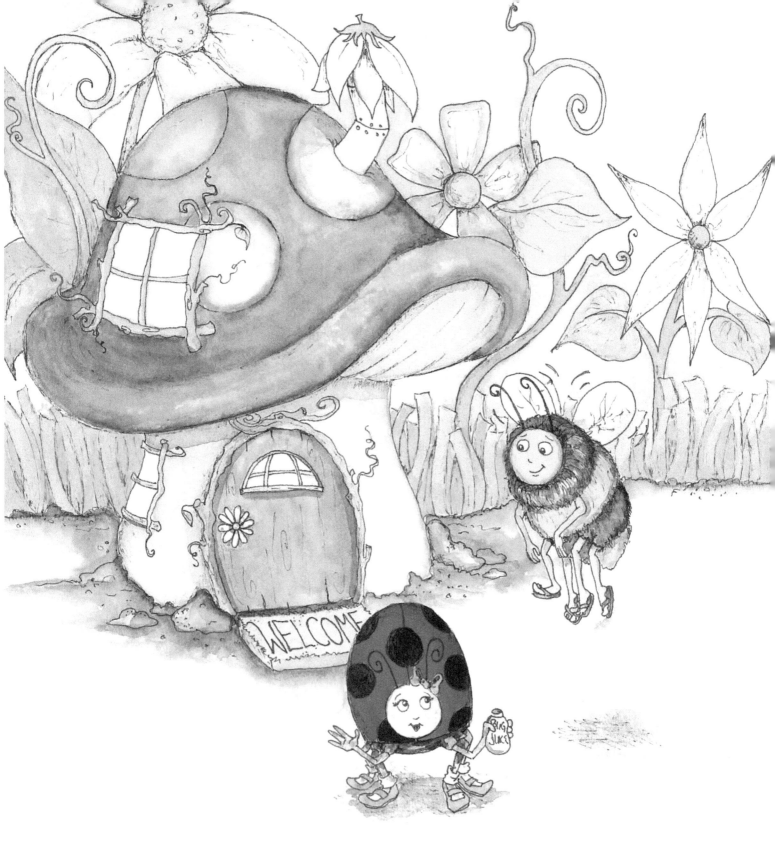

"Certainly a **BEEutiful** day!" said Lainy. "But,
Benny, you know I can't fly. I have never been strong enough.
Maybe we can walk together?"

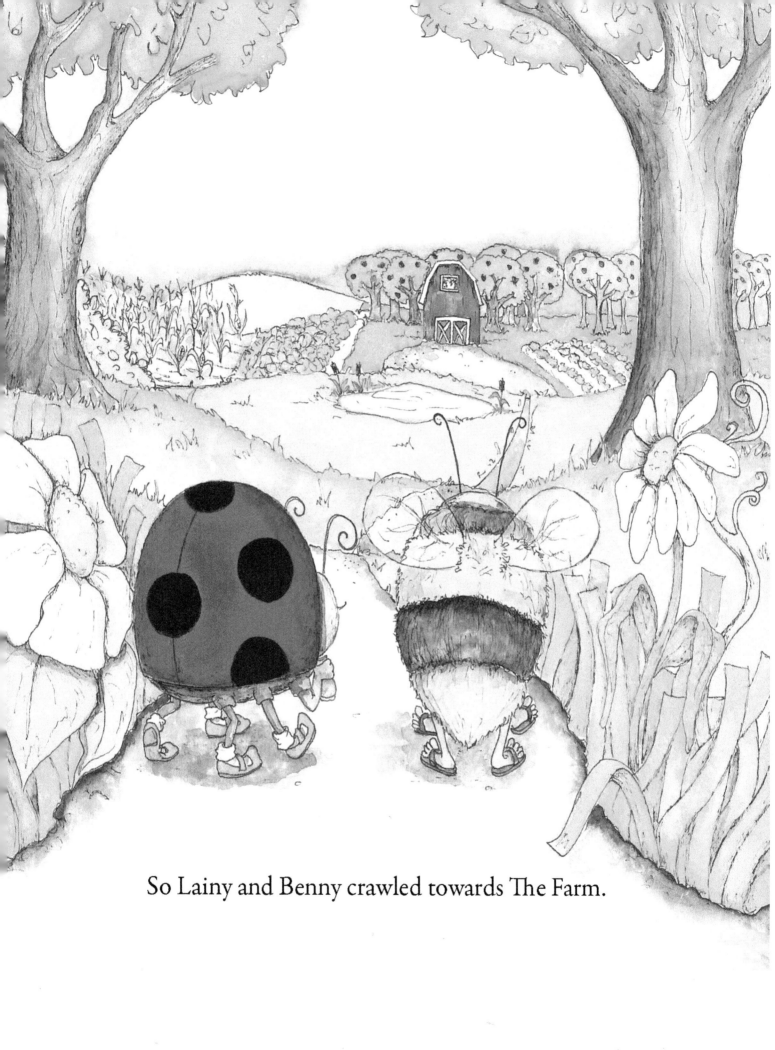

So Lainy and Benny crawled towards The Farm.

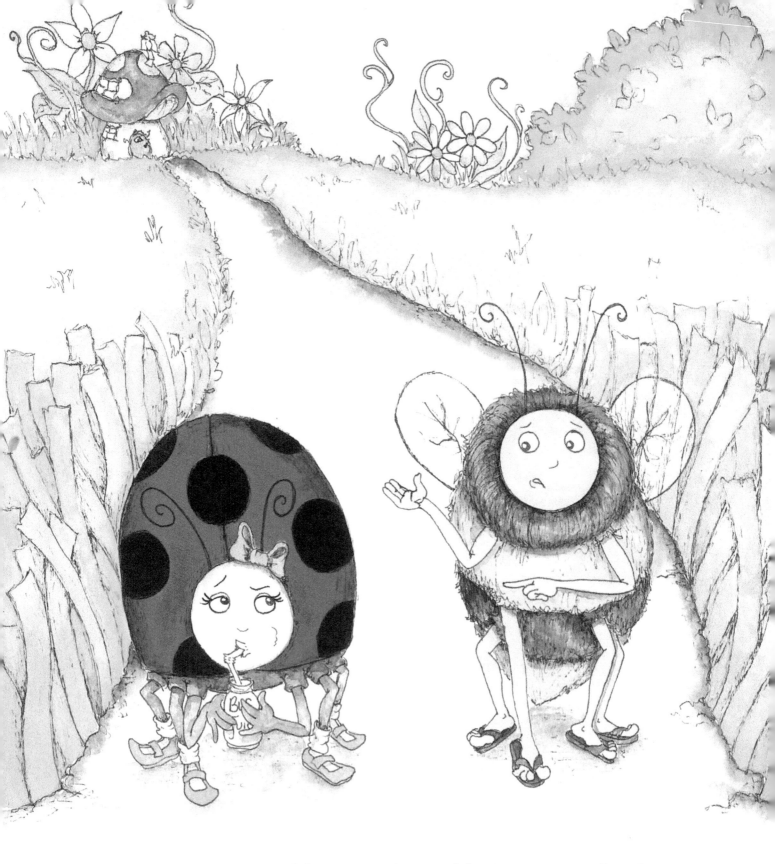

"Lainy, I've noticed how much you like Bug Juice. Don't you eat anything else?" asked Benny.

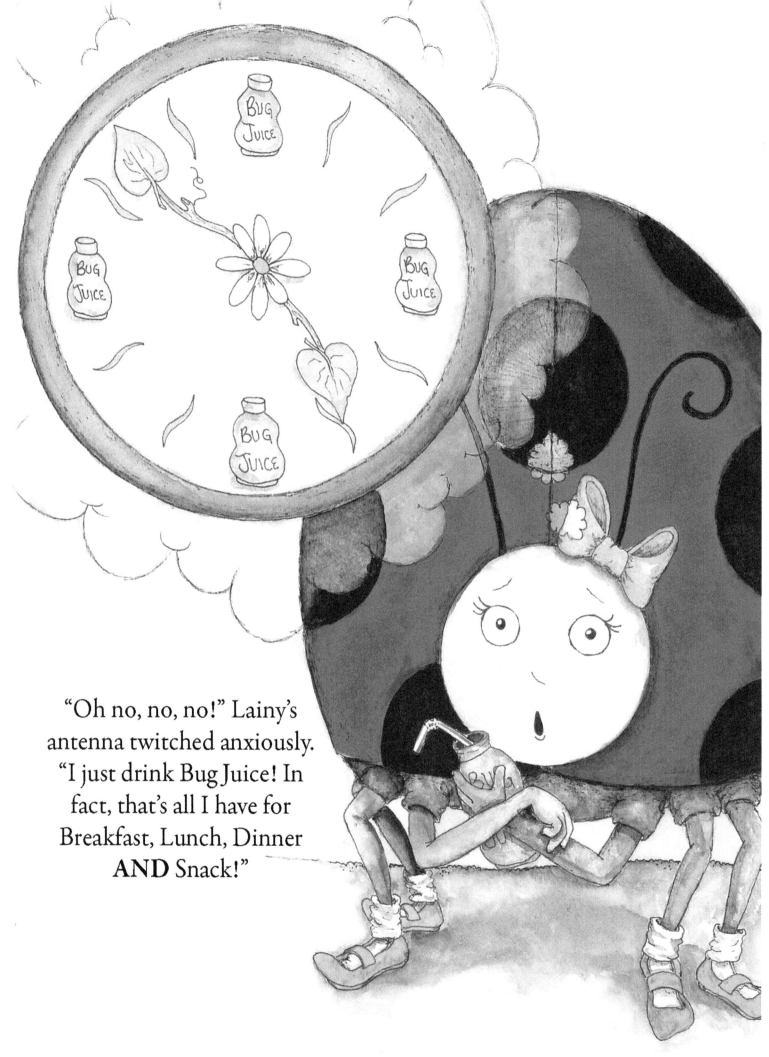

"Oh no, no, no!" Lainy's antenna twitched anxiously. "I just drink Bug Juice! In fact, that's all I have for Breakfast, Lunch, Dinner **AND** Snack!"

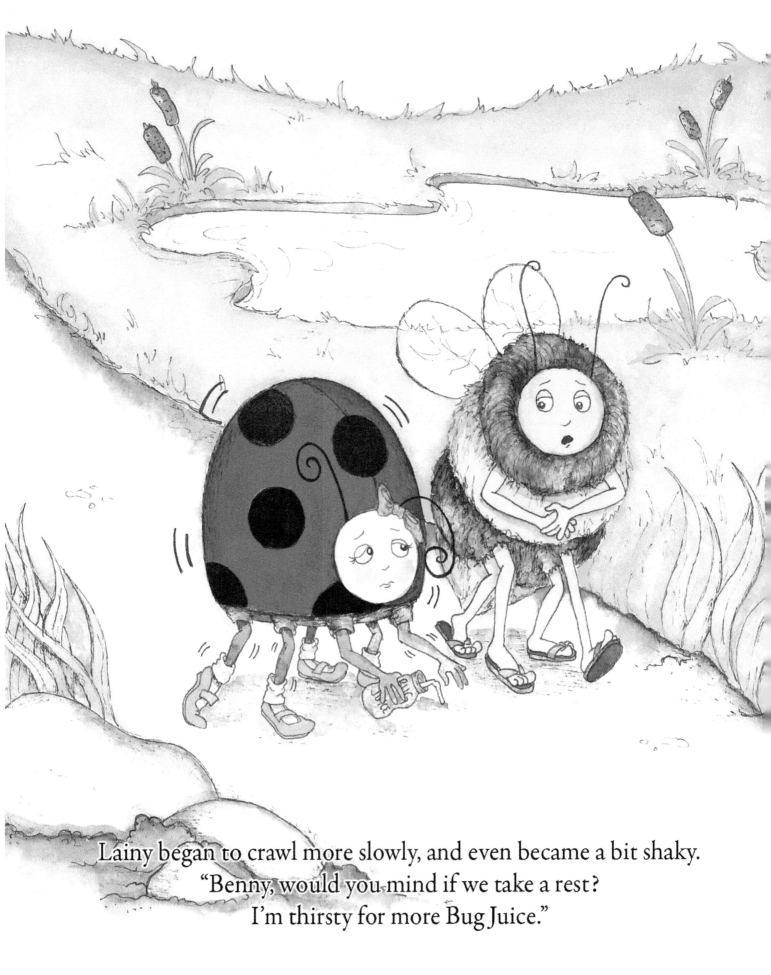

Lainy began to crawl more slowly, and even became a bit shaky.
"Benny, would you mind if we take a rest?
I'm thirsty for more Bug Juice."

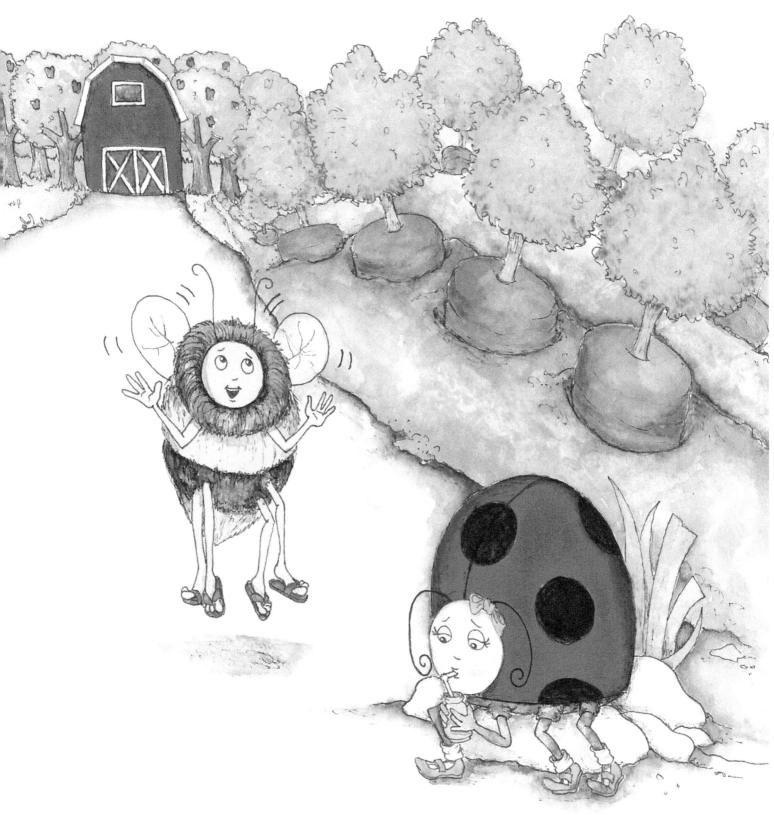

Benny buzzed around Lainy as she sipped her Bug Juice, and then they began to walk again.
Finally, they could see The Farm just ahead of them.

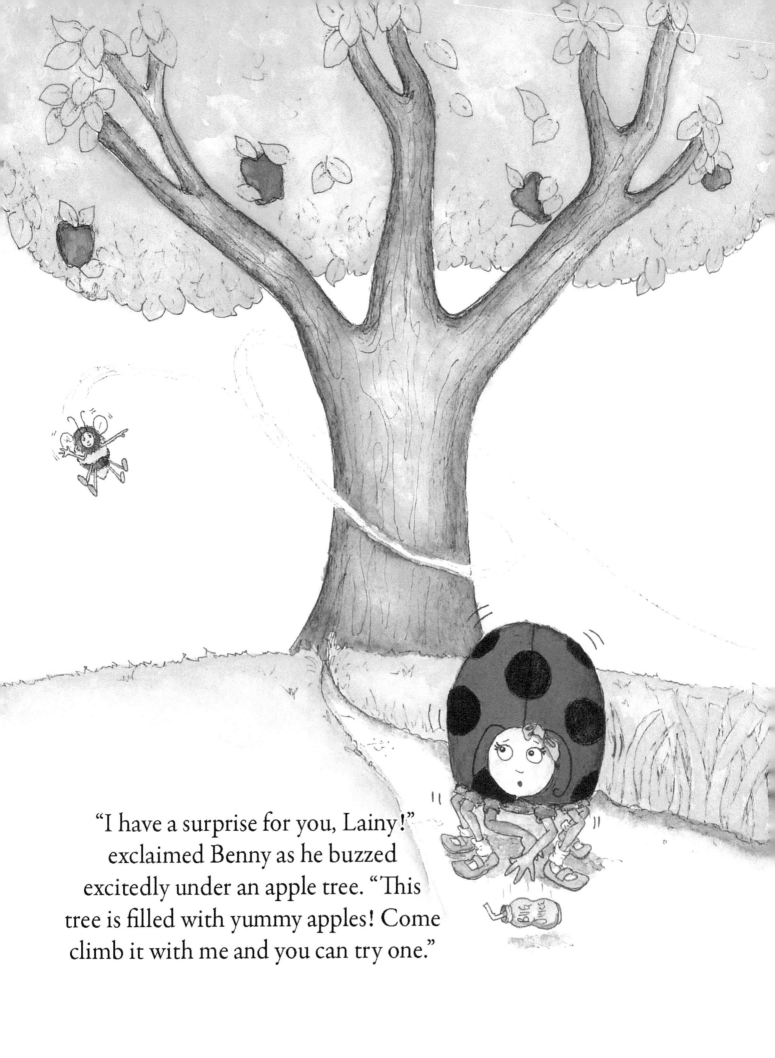

"I have a surprise for you, Lainy!" exclaimed Benny as he buzzed excitedly under an apple tree. "This tree is filled with yummy apples! Come climb it with me and you can try one."

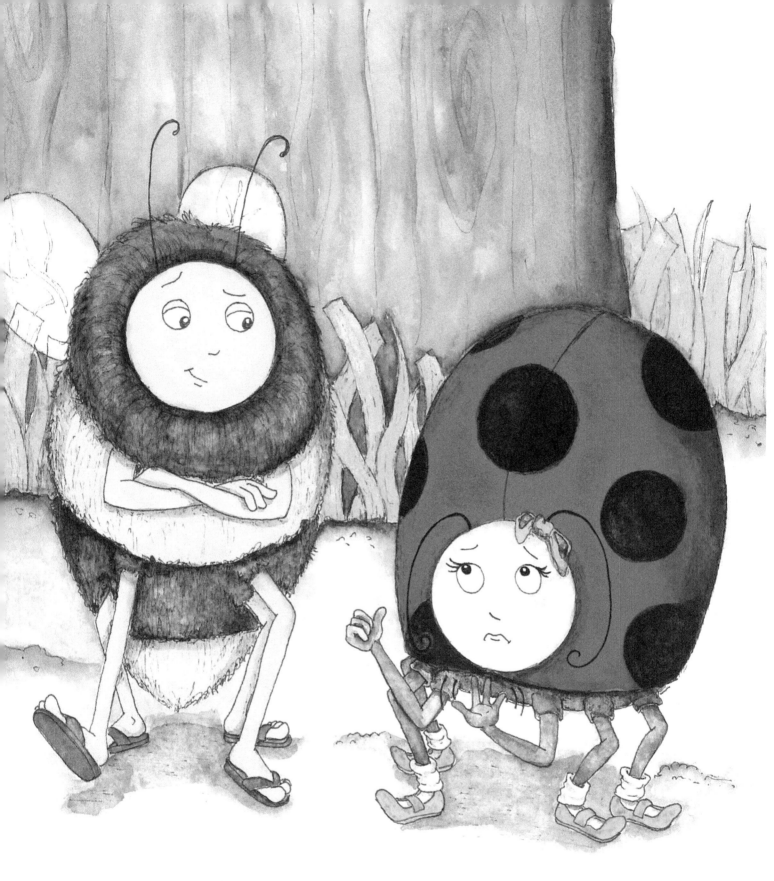

"Oh no, no, no!" replied Lainy, aghast.
"I **only** like my Bug Juice!"

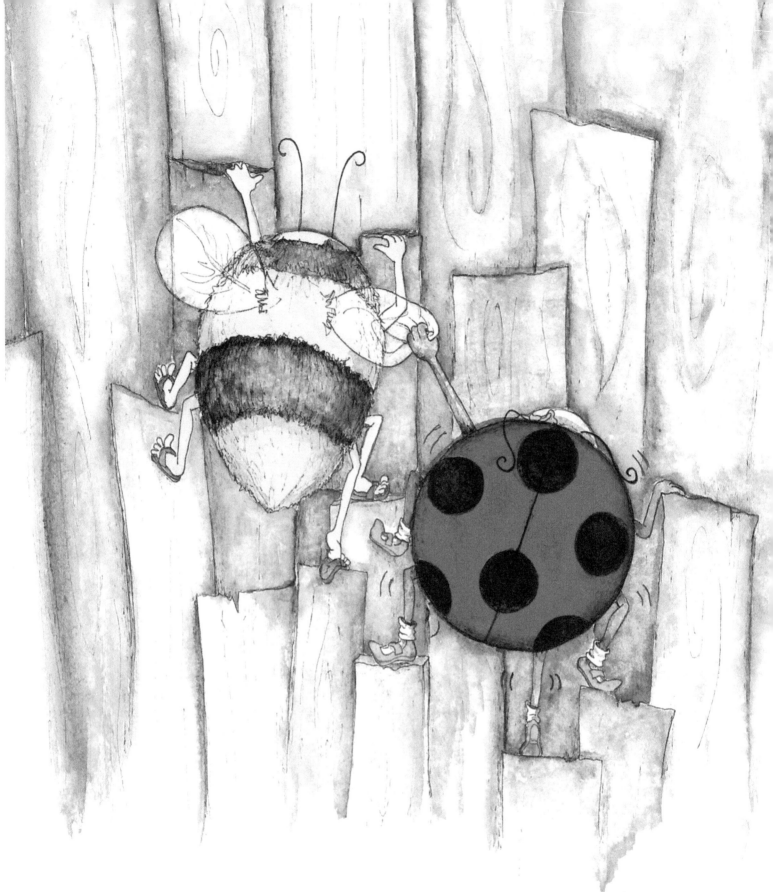

"Come – hold my wing – let's go up the tree together,"
encouraged Benny gently.

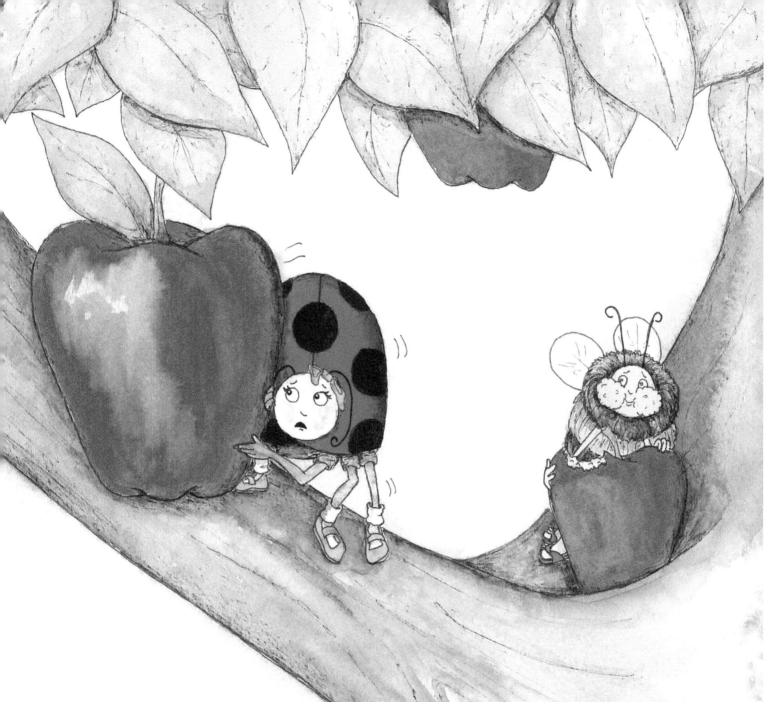

Before she knew it, Lainy was standing in front of a
big, juicy, red apple.
Benny took an enormous, crunchy bite and Lainy
watched as his wings fluttered happily.
"Pleeazzze try it... It's Buzzzilicious!" said Benny,
grinning and taking another crispy bite.
"**MMM**, sweet as honey!" he exclaimed.

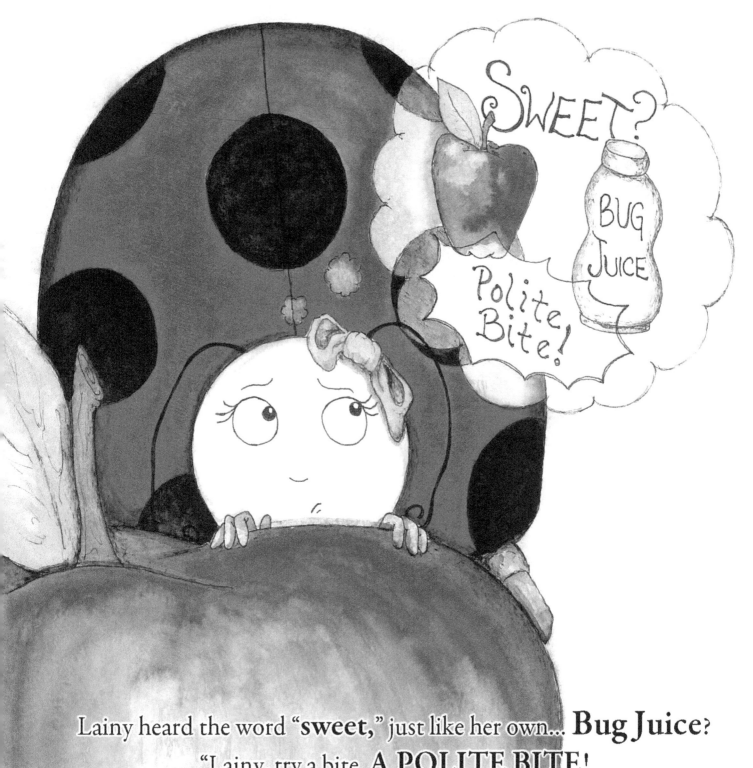

Lainy heard the word "**sweet**," just like her own... **Bug Juice**?
"Lainy, try a bite. **A POLITE BITE!**
A Polite Bite is just a small bite which allows you to taste
something you think you may not like. You can then decide if you
like that new food or not." said Benny.
"OK. For you, I will try a polite bite. Just this once," said Lainy.

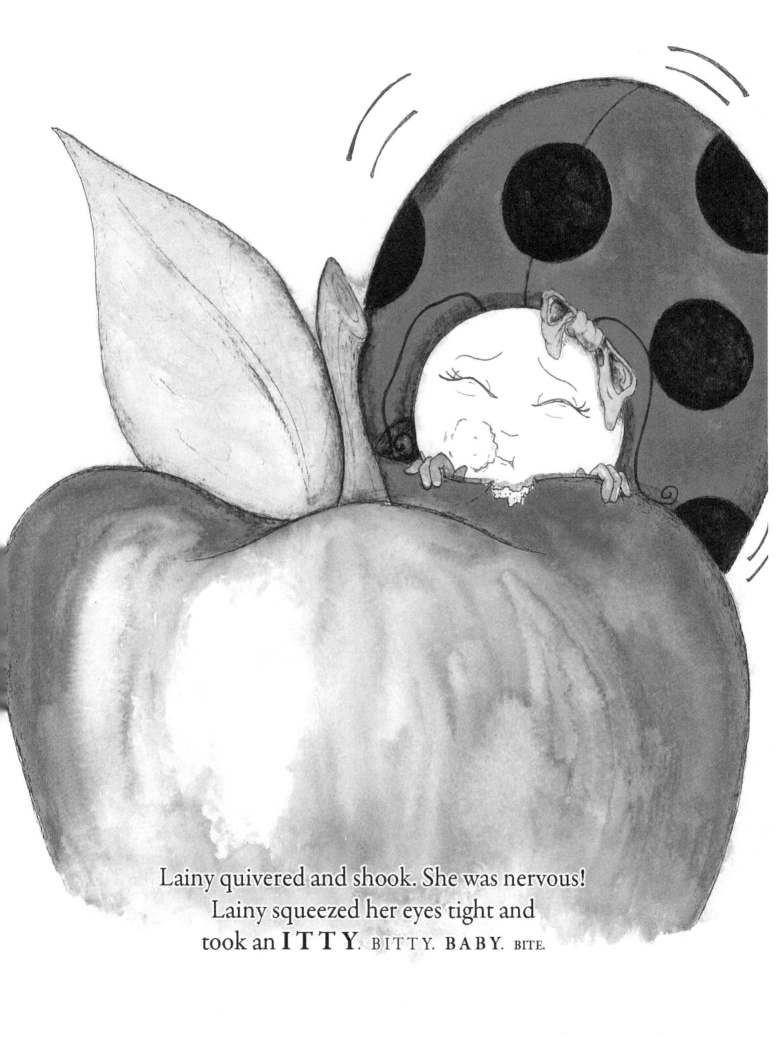

Lainy quivered and shook. She was nervous!
Lainy squeezed her eyes tight and
took an **ITTY**. BITTY. **BABY**. BITE.

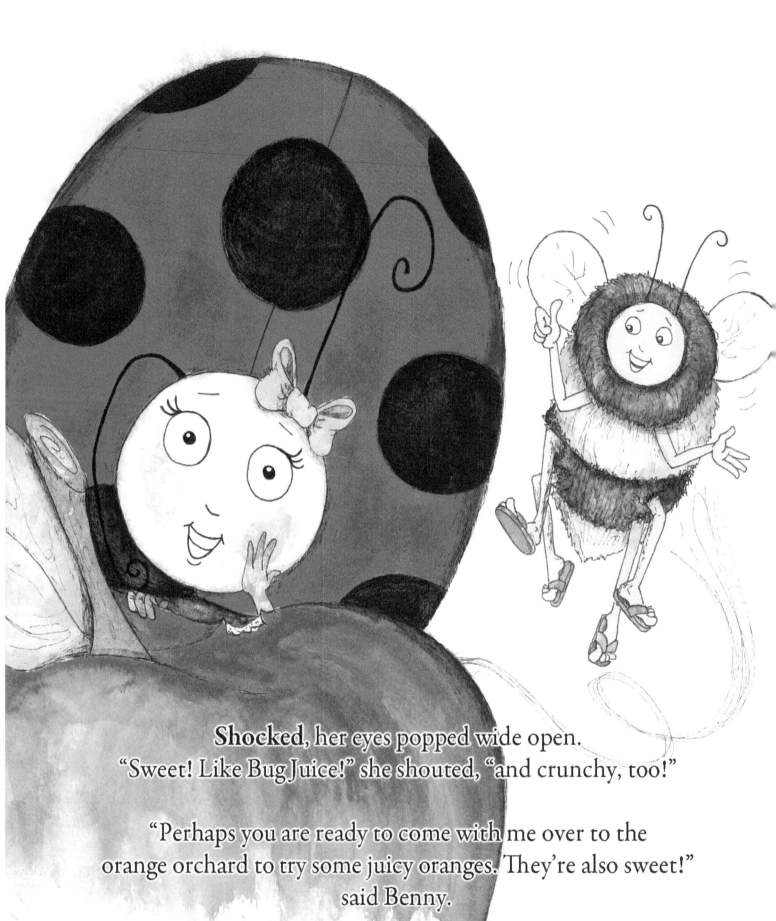

Shocked, her eyes popped wide open.
"Sweet! Like Bug Juice!" she shouted, "and crunchy, too!"

"Perhaps you are ready to come with me over to the
orange orchard to try some juicy oranges. They're also sweet!"
said Benny.

"OK, Benny, I trust you," muttered Lainy.

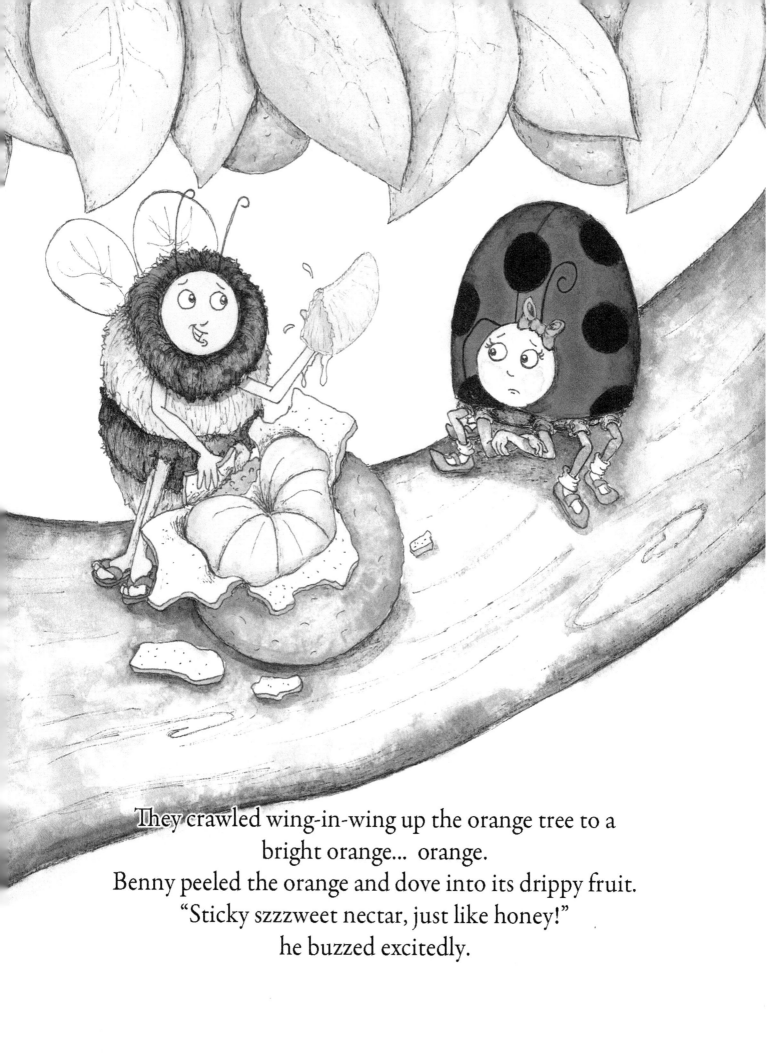

They crawled wing-in-wing up the orange tree to a
bright orange... orange.
Benny peeled the orange and dove into its drippy fruit.
"Sticky szzzweet nectar, just like honey!"
he buzzed excitedly.

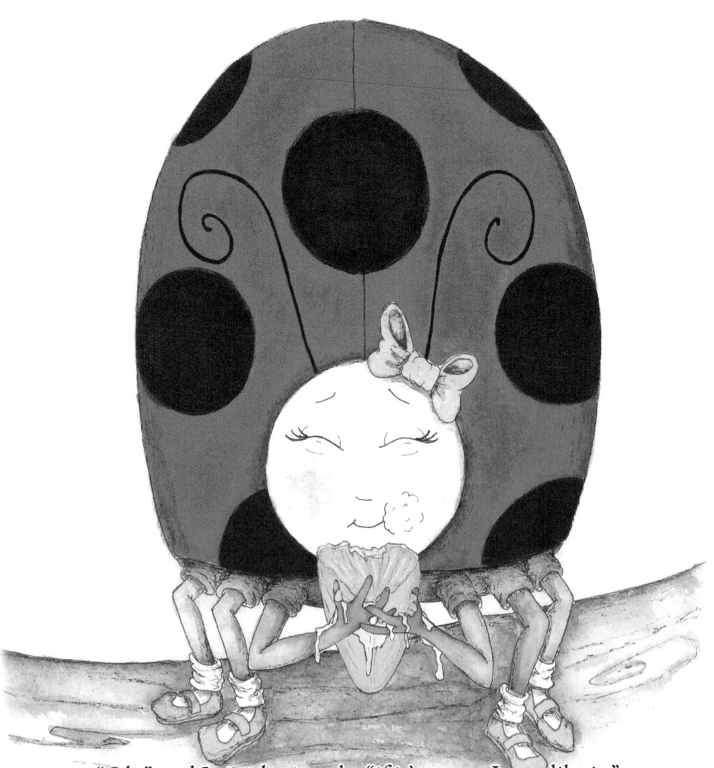

"Oh," said Lainy hesitantly, "if it's sweet, I may like it."
She nibbled a small section.
"Mmm, this is even juicier than Bug Juice! It's bright and zesty.
I think I like it as much as the crunchy, crispy apple!"

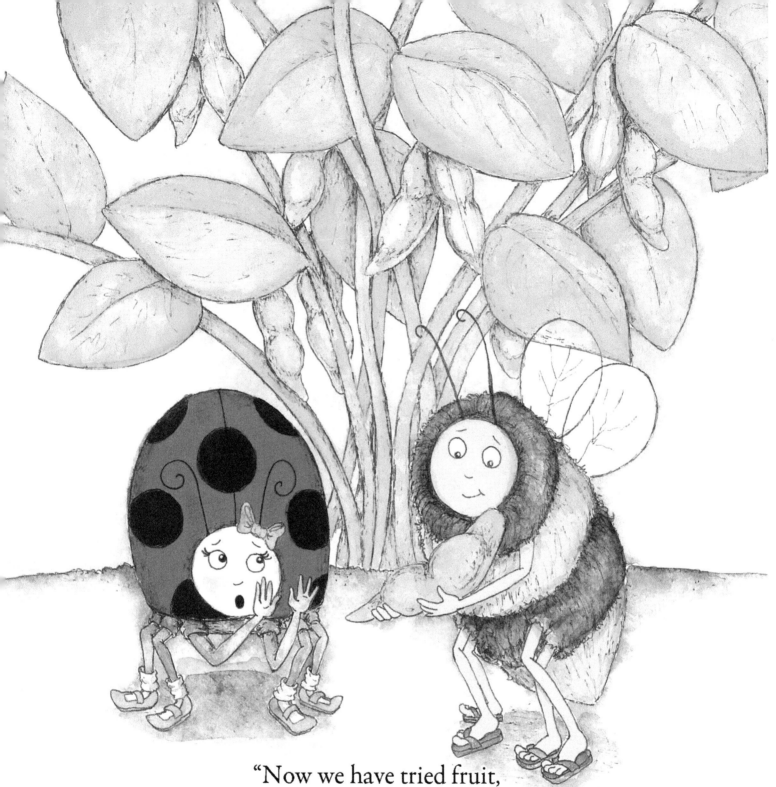

"Now we have tried fruit,
I want to show you my favorite vegetable," said Benny proudly. Benny
handed Lainy a bright green edamame pod.
"Pop one open and eat the pea," he encouraged.
"Oh, no, no, no! Nothing **G R E E N**!
No **G R E E N** foods! Green is **GROSS**!" groaned Lainy.

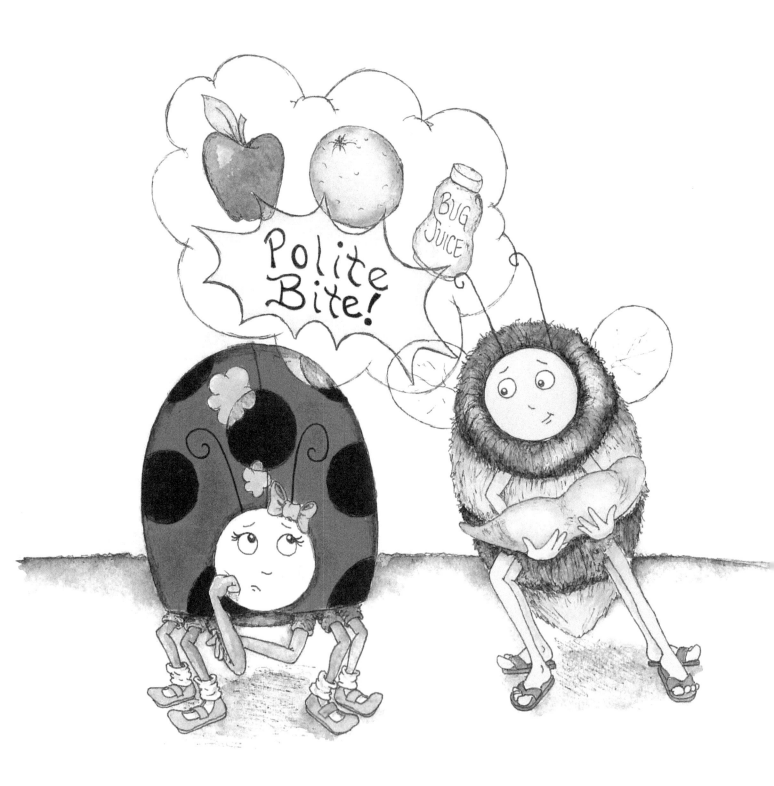

"Lainy, how do you know you don't like edamame if you have **NEVER** tried it? Remember the **POLITE BITE?**" smiled Benny.

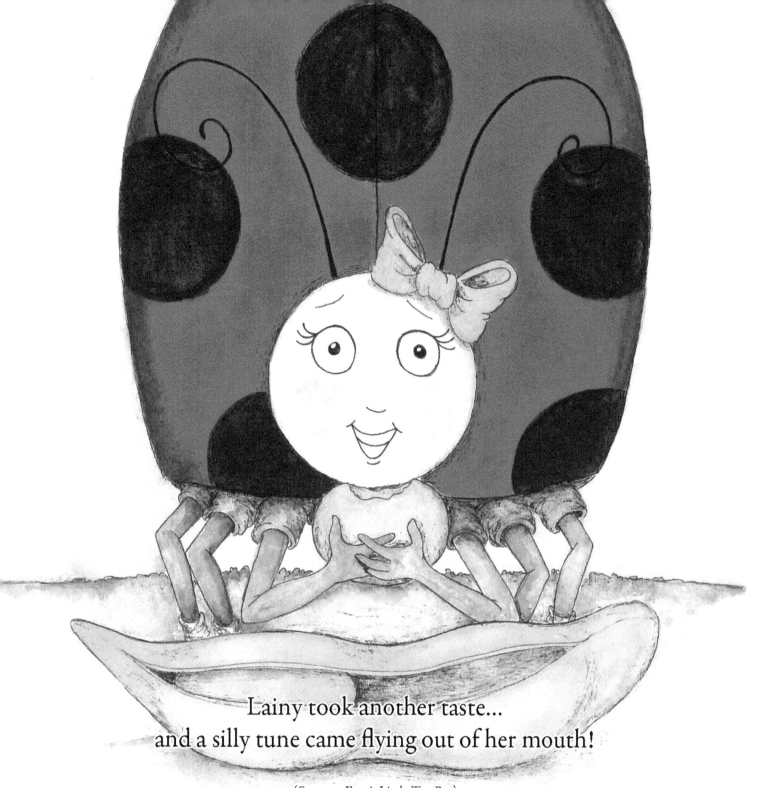

Lainy took another taste...
and a silly tune came flying out of her mouth!

(Sung to: I'm A Little Tea Pot)

Here's an edamame
Long and green
Here is the pod
And here are the beans
When I open each pod
Hear me scream
I want some more edamame beans!

Clap Clap

Yum Yum

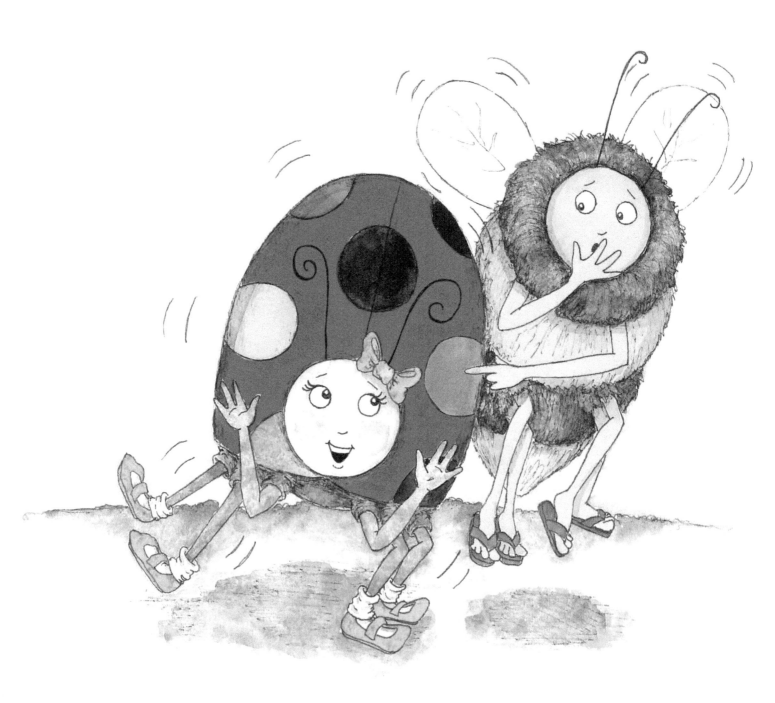

"Are you OK, Lainy? You are singing a silly song, your spots are changing color, and you look energized," observed Benny. "Goodness, I do feel buzzy Benny! Like you!" replied Lainy.

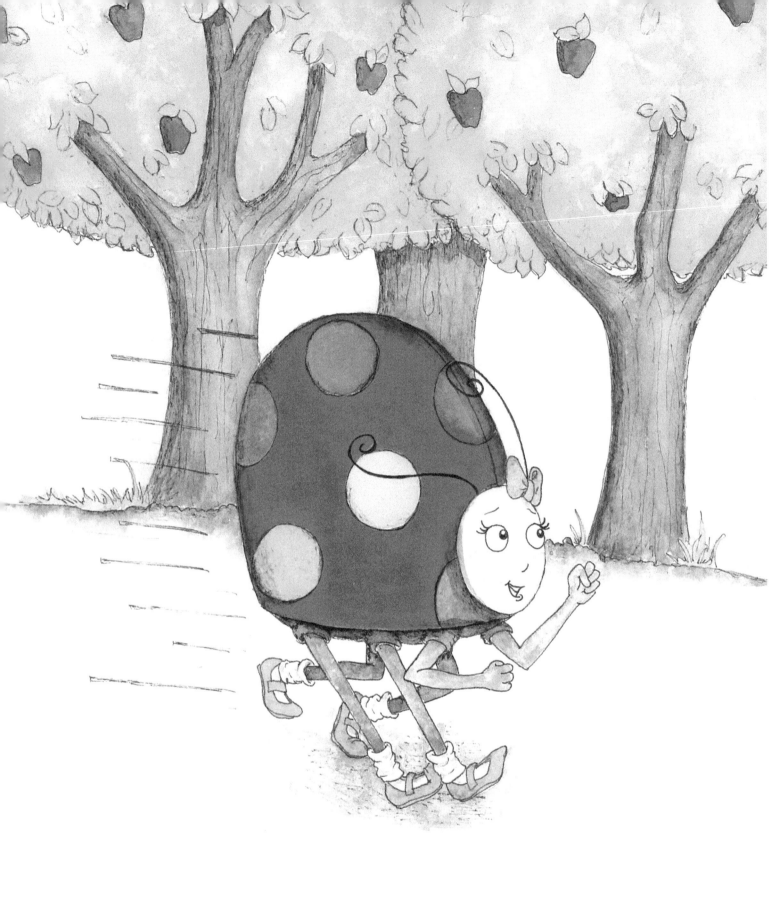

Without any warning, Lainy suddenly ran down the path and...

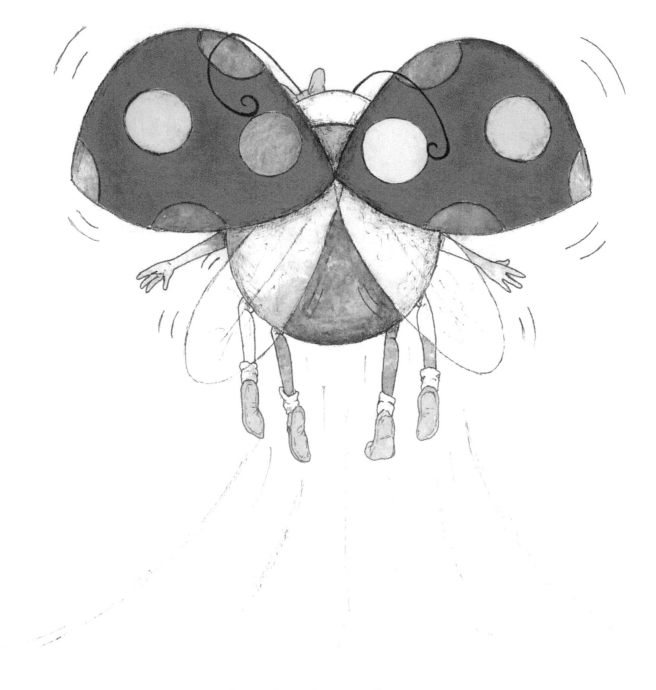

Took off into the air!

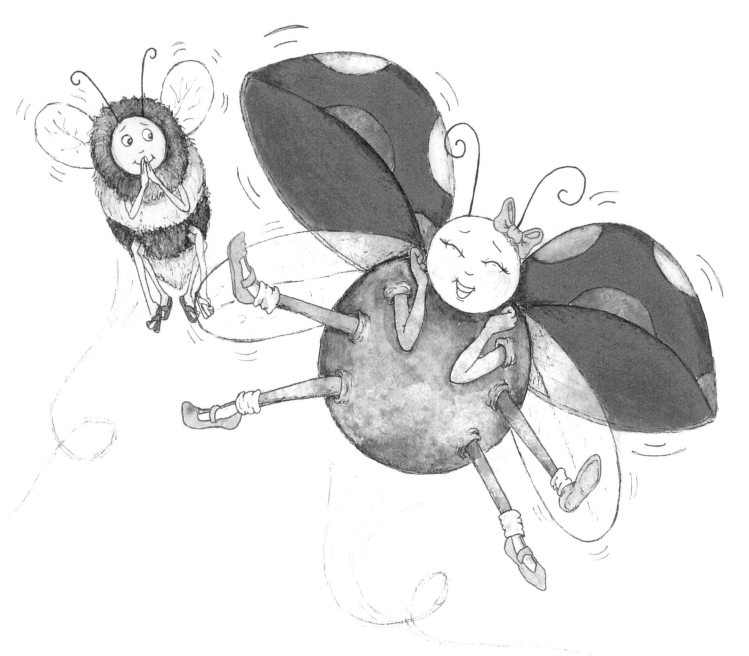

"Look Benny, I can **FLYYYYY!**
These new foods have hit just the right spots!"
Benny flew after Lainy. "Who would have thought?" he said, "You
not only tried new foods today, you gained enough energy to fly!"
Lainy was Polka-dot delighted.

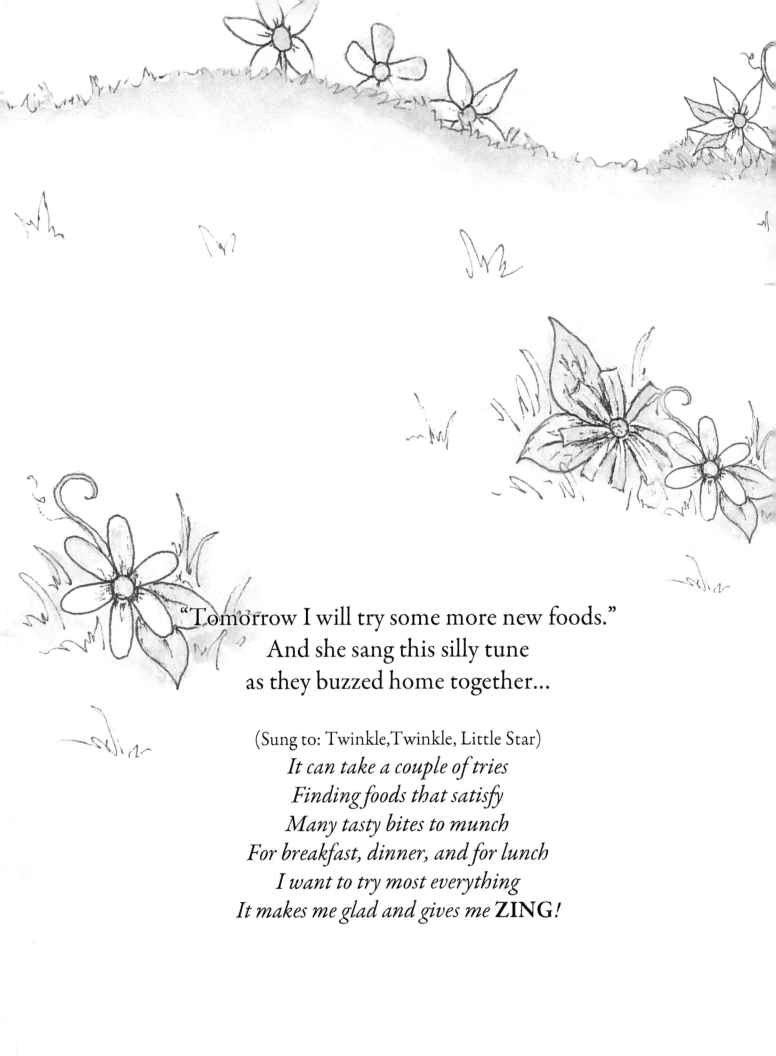

"Tomorrow I will try some more new foods."
And she sang this silly tune
as they buzzed home together...

(Sung to: Twinkle, Twinkle, Little Star)
It can take a couple of tries
Finding foods that satisfy
Many tasty bites to munch
For breakfast, dinner, and for lunch
I want to try most everything
It makes me glad and gives me **ZING!**

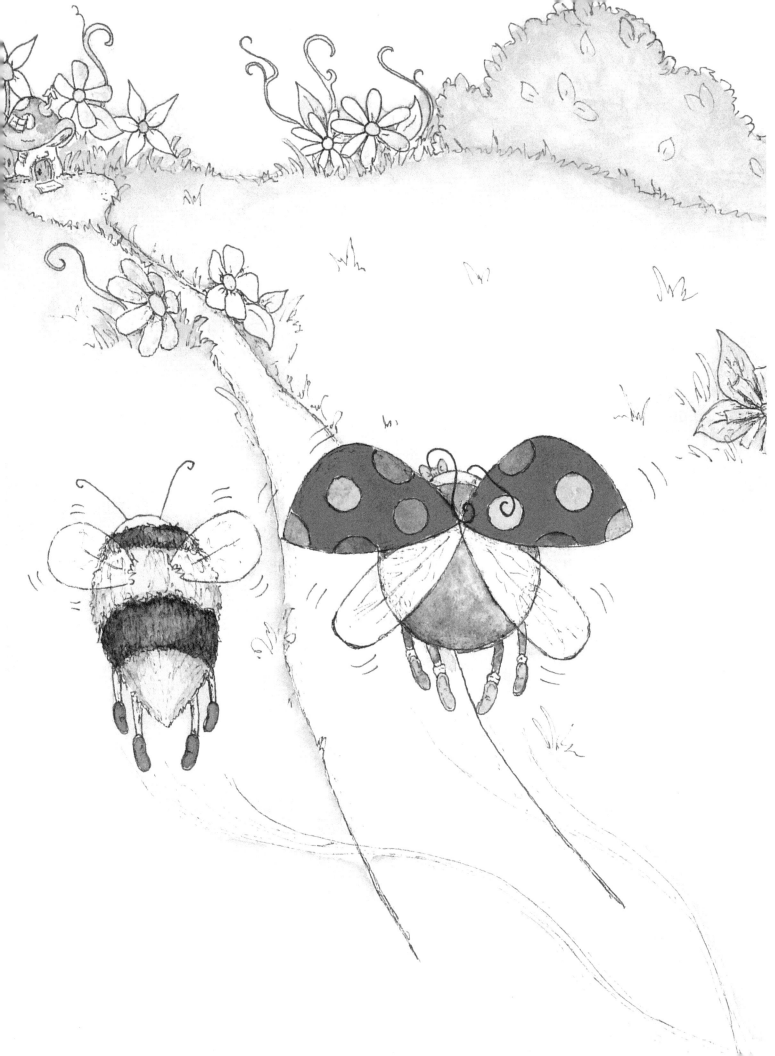

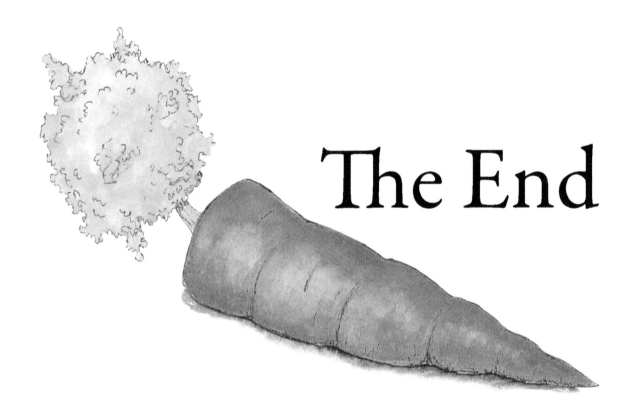

The End

Lainy's Ladybug Recipe

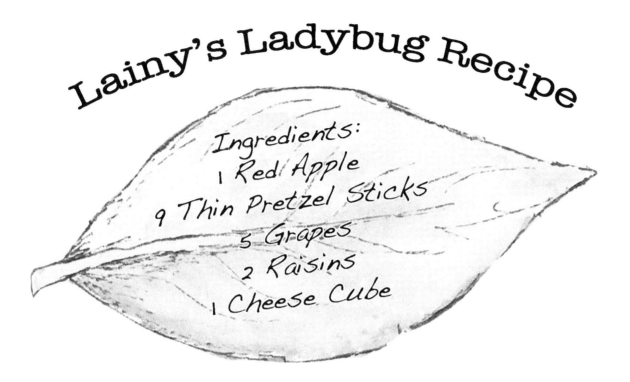

Ingredients:
1 Red Apple
9 Thin Pretzel Sticks
5 Grapes
2 Raisins
1 Cheese Cube

Slice apples in half from top to bottom and scoop out the cores using a knife or melon baller. Place each apple half flat side down on a small plate or napkin.

Take three pretzel sticks and break them in half, press five pretzels into the back of the apple and press one in the front where the head should be.

Once the pretzel sticks are placed in the apple take five grapes and stick one grape on each pretzel to form Lainy's spots.

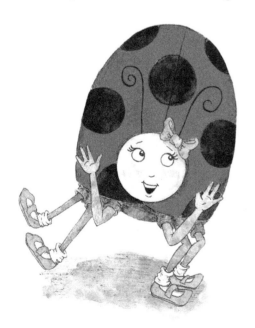

Take the cheese cube and place it on the final pretzel stick at the front of the apple for Lainy's head.

Now take four more pretzel sticks and press them into the apple to form four legs.

Once the legs have been placed, take the final two pretzel sticks and press one end of the remaining two pretzels into the two raisins. Press the other end of the pretzel into the apple to form the antennae.

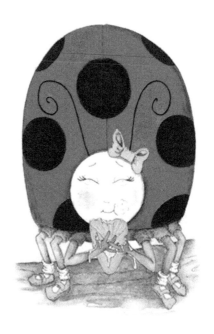

About the Author

Emma J. Fogt dreamed up Lainy Ladybug in 2001 supported by a grant from the Delaware Valley Chapter of the Society of Nutrition Education. Emma is a Registered Dietitian/Nutritionist, Consultant & Entrepreneur and lives in the woods of Pennsylvania with her husband, two grown children and joyful Labradoodle.

About the Illustrator

Lori B. Wicks has been drawing ever since she could hold a pencil. She feels extremely blessed to now be able to use her talent to help bring authors' visions to life. Lori lives on a farm in Kansas with her husband and 5 year old son.

CPSIA information can be obtained at www.ICGtesting.com
Printed in the USA
LVOW05s1056080315

429456LV00003B/8/P